Shit
ISN'T A
DIRTY
WORD

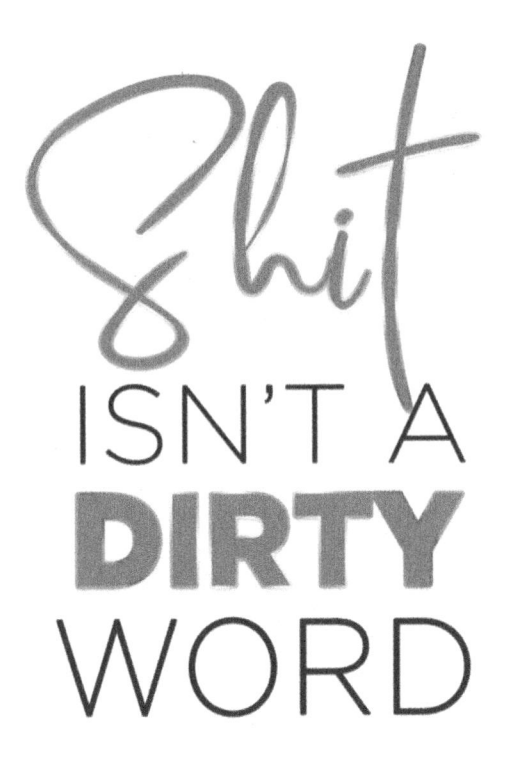

An Unorthodox Approach to Colon and Digestive Health

KARIN NAHMANI

HOUSECAPACITY

Copyright © 2021 by Karin Nahamani

All rights reserved. No part of this publication may be reproduced, distributed, or transmitted in any form or by any means, including photocopying, recording, or other electronic or mechanical methods, without the prior written permission of the publisher, except in the case of brief quotations embodied in critical reviews and certain other noncommercial uses permitted by copyright law. For permission requests, write to the publisher, addressed "Attention: Permissions Coordinator," at the address below.

House Capacity Publishing
support@housecapacity.com
www.housecapacity.com

Printed in the United States of America

ISBN-13: 978-1-955649-01-8

Shit Isn't a Dirty Word

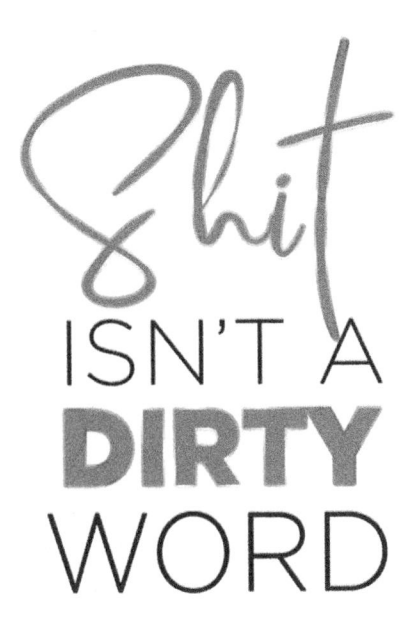

An Unorthodox Approach to Colon and Digestive Health

KARIN NAHMANI

	Intro	7
1	The Shit Whisperer	9
2	What Is a Colonic and Why Do I Need One?	13
3	The Good, The Bad, and the Bacteria	19
4	But Is It Gonna Hurt?	23
5	They Still Wanted to Poison Me	29
6	My Husband & I Could Not Get Pregnant	35
7	A Spiritual Cleanse	41
8	The Scoop on Poop	47
9	Health, Wellness, And Tasty Tidbits	55
10	Other Forms of Detox	63
Epilogue	Marching Orders!	67
Afterword	Genita M. Mason H.H.P., N.C., F.E	69

CRAP, Poop, **DUNG**, BM, manure, *FECES*, *take a dump*, **malarkey**, Droppings, excrement, *HOOEY*, *turd*, number two, **DEFECATION**, *poo*, **STOOL**, SCAG, *bach*, **ROTH**, CODSWALLOP, BUNK, *buncombe* ...

*A*t the end of the day, when all is said and done, and when nature calls, it's all just a bunch of **SHIT**! But we shouldn't be afraid to talk about it!

We all do it; some more than others, but "it" happens. My goal with this book, among other things, is to break the taboo of talking about what nature intended us to do, and that's get rid of waste and toxins. We have to call it something, and whether that be taking a dump, going potty or simply shitting, it's perfectly natural. Certainly, men can often be more comfortable about discussing it than women, but it's nothing to be ashamed of, especially if you're having difficulty. Your doctor has seen and heard it all, and as someone who administers colonics for a living, there's nothing I haven't seen.

Despite many segments of this book having a light-hearted approach, I take one's health and wellness very seriously. Think about this: By not being ashamed to discuss irregular bowel habits, being constipated, or a whole variety of other issues related to "shit," just might save your life or someone you love! Isn't that worth it?

1

THE SHIT WHISPERER

I've been affectionally referred to as the "Ass Doctor," "Butt Doctor" and "The Shit Whisperer." My name is Karin Nahmani and I'm a certified colon hydrotherapist, naturopathic doctor, massage therapist and doula. A doula is a birth companion, coach and supporter before, during and/or after childbirth.

I am also the proud mother of four and married to an incredible, supportive man. I'm originally from Israel and initially wanted to become a medical doctor, but I quickly realized that wasn't for me. It would take years and years to finish and I was too impatient for that. Even though I did begin my studies, I soon put that aside after speaking with my sister who worked for the University of Natural Health. She thought maybe I should study reflexology. "But I don't like touching people's feet!" She still encouraged me to pursue it, because I liked to help people and heal them. It was a year long course and after a while, I decided I would look into massage therapy. But to be honest, at this point in my life, I was still trying to find myself.

My sister suggested that I should go the naturopathic route; which essentially is an all-natural approach to healing. A naturopathic doctor uses reflexology, Shiatsu massage, ideology, herbology, homeopathic treatments and it promotes self-healing by finding out the cause of one's health problems, not just treating the symptoms like most western medicine is practiced. I liked this direction. I could be a licensed doctor in four years and begin healing, whereas a traditional medical doctor would take ten years or more. It seemed to be the right path for me. I thoroughly enjoyed what I was doing, and I was good at it!

My nutritional instructor was the pioneer of colonics in Israel. To finish my required hours, she offered me an opportunity to volunteer in her clinic and teach me how to administer colonics. I was volunteering one week when cancer patients came in to receive colonics, massage and reflexology. When I saw the smiles on their faces after their treatments; I knew this was what I wanted to do!

To say I got into colonic hydrotherapy through the "back door" would be very accurate.

To say I got into colonic hydrotherapy through the "back door" would be very accurate. My goal was to treat cancer patients with everything I knew. To this day, my dream is to open a cancer clinic and help everyone I can. I don't know when this will come to be, but I know it will happen.

I was doing well in Israel, working at a clinic. Unfortunately my personal life wasn't as good. I needed a break. I called a friend in the

United States and we planned a trip for me to come to Los Angeles for three months.

I was still very involved with my college and the director of the school told me I still needed to complete my internship if I was to get my naturopathic degree. I told him I would return after the three months to do so. He suggested I contact a friend of his in L.A. who owned a massage school and if I interned there, he would sign off on my internship hours.

At the time, no one knew much about the health benefits of massage. Even to this day, many only think of massage as for pleasure at a spa. I began teaching two classes a day, six days a week. My three months in L.A. had become just over two years.

I had more than 300 amazing students who learned nutrition, reflexology, therapeutic massage and pregnancy massage. At the same time, I was also giving colonics. This was in 2001 and back then colonics weren't well known. And if it was, it was kept very private. No one was comfortable talking about it. That's something I've always wanted to change.

I worked for a chiropractor and it was a fantastic experience until about 2006 when I decided I didn't want to work for others, I wanted to open my own clinic. I was gambling on myself and going to start my own business.

My husband helped me find a space through a contact of his on Sunset Boulevard in Hollywood. Although everything seemed to fall into place, we were heading into a recession here in the U.S. and it wasn't the most logical time to open a clinic offering colonics. But that wasn't going to stop me!

There were five other clinics in the Los Angeles area and I knew all of them. I was the newbie. No one, other than a few clients, knew who I was. The other clinics were advertising in newspapers, gay magazines, you name it. But everyone around me, including my husband were skeptical "Who's going to get a colonic? No one knows you!" All I could say was, "They will!"

And the word spread. I did do a little bit of advertising, but word of mouth is by far the best way to get new clients. And one after another started coming. I had a good reputation and was getting a great deal or referrals. My first year I had over 1000 clients! It was magical. I couldn't believe it.

I've helped so many people in the twenty years I've been providing healthy, healing services and my goal is reach out to many more so they too can learn that Shit Isn't A Dirty Word!

2

WHAT IS A COLONIC AND WHY DO I NEED ONE?

Colonic.
High Colonic.
Hydro-Colonic Therapy.
Colon Hydro Therapy.
Colon Cleanse.
Colon Irrigation.

A colonic is the deep cleaning of your colon with warm, filtered water and nothing else. No stimulants; which is what's in most laxatives. No glycerin or oils—nothing but water. And it is not an enema, which really only does superficial cleaning of rectum and lower portion of the colon.

You could be thinking: "I'm a healthy person. I try to eat well, exercise and take care of myself. Why would I need a colonic?" You might be all of that, but it doesn't mean you're still not full of shit! Healthy people still need colonics. Everyone needs a colonic from time to time. Some more than others; some more frequently than others; it all depends on the person.

> **You might be all of that, but it doesn't mean you're still not full of shit!**

There are numerous reasons your colon gets clogged, not just poor nutrition or lifestyle. Stress is a huge factor and in today's hectic world, we're all stressed out. Anxiety is also a big source. Gas can cause the waste to stick and not release. And "holding it" or not going when you should, is a huge problem.

As small children our colons are at peak efficiency. We eat, we poop. Our young lives are typically stress free, with perhaps a little bit of gas now and again, but otherwise we are a well-oiled pooping machine. But as we get older and the everyday stresses of life, we start to eat foods we shouldn't, we start taking medications for our various ailments, we drink alcohol; a whole variety of factors and waste ends up sticking around in our colon. Parents suggesting their kids "hold it" when they need to go, is not a good idea. Our bodies tell us when it's time to eliminate and when we don't, when we hold it, we're essentially forcing ourselves to become constipated.

And then the embarrassment factor.

Going "number two," "taking a dump," "pooping," "dropping a deuce"; is all a very natural thing. Many people are uncomfortable using public restrooms and end up "holding it" for many hours until they get back home and can go in private. Couples who have been married for years won't "go" when the other is around, once again causing constipation. It's nothing to be ashamed about, but many people are.

This is one taboo I don't associate with. My husband says I have no shame when it comes to going to the restroom and he's right! I've tried to instill that with my children as well. When you have to go, you go. I've told each of their school teachers that if they ask to use the restroom they are allowed to right away.

When we hold it, we're causing our colons to become clogged. When you're constipated and you eat, you further exasperate the situation. Most meat takes at least twenty-four hours to fully digest, dairy products take about eight to ten hours. Meanwhile, if you're still constipated, what you've just eaten causes you gas, bloating, decreased energy levels and discomfort. Over time the built up waste not only hides in the pockets of your colon, but it can turn into plaque. And this can lead to health problems. This is why you need a colonic.

Like a plumber unclogging your drain, a colonic unclogs your colon. I'm going to walk you through a typical colonic experience. During the procedure, I'm pushing sometimes as much as two gallons of water through your colon. Don't worry, I'm not doing it all at once!

> **Like a plumber unclogging your drain, a colonic unclogs your colon.**

First, with your help, I gently insert a lubricated, sterile & disposable speculum into your rectum. A rectal speculum is a small device that is inserted into the anus to keep the anus open for diagnostic viewing of the rectum, for anal surgery and for administering a colonic.

Attached to the speculum is a small tube for the incoming water and a larger tube for the waste to travel through into the FDA-registered Hydro San Plus (closed system), which allows waste material to be eliminated through the instrument and out the drain line without odor.

The incoming water is filtered and at about 100 degrees Fahrenheit (38 Celsius). By the time it pushes into your colon it will be very close to your body temperate. You'll barely even feel it at first. Then as the colon beings to fill, you'll start to feel the urge to "go." There might be a little bit of temporary discomfort before we release, but it's rarely even the slightest bit painful.

This is all done in a private room. You'll be wearing a hospital-type gown and resting comfortably, face up on a table with a warm blanket over you. We can even listen to music if you like.

As I gently push water into your colon from the inside, I'm lightly massaging your colon from the outside helping to loosen and release built up waste and perhaps some trapped gas. You and I can see what is being released via clear tubes. There is no smell and it is very hygienic and sanitary. And then I repeat the process by gently pushing more water and continue with the massage. The more that's released, the farther into the colon I can push water, further releasing more and more waste.

The water actually moves through the ascending, transverse and descending colon within seconds. What takes time is filling the colon, which acts like a balloon and slowly expands. We're not pushing water as far as the intestines; perhaps a tiny bit might make it that far, but the intestines are part of the digestive system and we're not cleaning that.

After digestion, the waste is delivered to the colon. Through a normal bowel movement, waste is eliminated; but not necessarily all of it. Through years or poor diet, poor nutrition, preservatives in our food, everyday stress and so forth, the fecal matter and toxins end up sticking to the walls to the colon. Even a relatively healthy forty-year-old person can have as much as twenty or more years of waste sitting in the colon. That affects your health. That affects how you feel. Maybe not now, but eventually it will. Through a proper colonic, that built-up waste is removed and you'll begin to feel the positive affects of being "clean" on the inside.

The colon consists of little pockets and that's where the waste will stick. When we introduce the water, it loosens and releases that stuck waste. A laxative can't do that and if used regularly, is actually harmful since it's using a stimulant to force you to go. Whereas a colonic actually helps the colon to become stronger and more efficient.

Health and wellness begins in the gut. Years and years ago a grandmother or mother would treat a fever, a headache, sickness, you name it, with an enema. They instinctively knew that the waste within our bodies was what was causing our illness. And when the inside is clean, the outside reflects that. We simply feel and look better.

Trust me on this. With regular colonic therapy you'll no longer be full of shit and you'll start to look and feel amazing!

3

The Good, The Bad, and the Bacteria

I hear it all the time, especially from doctors, "Colonics are bad because they wash out the good bacteria." To that I say, "Big deal! Of course they do." The problem is that the good bacteria (acidophilus, bifidus to name a few) which is the flora inside our gut that helps with digestion and keeping us healthy by removing toxins and turning them into waste–our little soldiers; but when they aren't treated right, with a poor diet and too much or unnecessary medications, they can't do their jobs and become or "go bad."

After a colonic, I always recommend my clients take probiotic supplements. Which contain billions of good bacteria to replenish what was washed out. You can also find probiotics in yogurt, kimchi and a whole variety of healthy foods. This keeps our gut in check and working properly.

Once we reach about twelve years old our bodies no longer know how to create healthy bacteria, so we need to treat our bodies properly with nutrition and supplements to keep our insides healthy. When we don't, we get the flu and other illnesses because our immune system, which starts in the gut, is compromised. Other symptoms of an unhealthy gut are low energy, gas and bloating, restless sleep, bad skin; the list goes on. But it doesn't stop there.

Every single minute of every single day, doctors are prescribing medications which are killing our good bacteria and making our guts unhealthy; which may cause us to become constipated. Then the same doctor will prescribe a laxative, which is a stimulant, and what does it do? It washes away the good bacteria and we're right back where we started.

Don't get me wrong, I think there are many amazing medical doctors out there saving lives every day. There really are. But I hope one day that these doctors start to see their patients as people, as individuals, not just an object that needs to be treated, medicated and sent home. There is a lot more to health and wellness than doing it by the numbers. And instead of treating the symptom, how about we prevent the problem from happening in the first place? And definitely don't make it worse by killing all of the good bacteria that we so desperately need to keep us healthy.

> **Come to me for a colonic because you want to – not because you have to.**

I tell so many people, come to me for a colonic because you want to – not because you have to.

If we get rid of the bad stuff inside you, then we can prevent illnesses from happening; we prevent you from getting sick, from feeling bad and ending up at a medical doctor's office in need of medications or worse, in the hospital because you didn't take care of yourself. This may seem dramatic, but it's very true. Keep your body clean, treat it well and you'll be amazed at how good you look and feel.

The colon is approximately 5.7 feet long. Yes, 5.7 feet of shit! You can potentially have as much as fifteen pounds of waste in your colon. Yes, fifteen POUNDS! I shit you not! And it can be very, very old. Which means toxins from maybe ten or more years ago are sitting inside your body and affecting your health. You wouldn't go ten years without changing the oil in your car, why would you want nasty, old gunk in your body for that same amount of time?

A positive side effect of colonics is weight loss. Not to say you have colonics to lose weight per se, but if we washed out fifteen pounds of waste, well you'll have lost fifteen pounds of body weight. But it's not fat, it's shit! However, when you get rid of the waste, then your body becomes more efficient and in turn you can more easily lose weight with a healthy lifestyle because you're clean! Clean and efficient on the inside.

When you're clean, you feel good. You have energy and you'll want to burn that energy and guess what? You'll lose weight.

Think of when you just did a deep cleaning of your house, you don't want anyone tracking mud inside or messing it up, right? Same goes after a colonic, you're nice and clean and you won't want to put anything bad inside to make it dirty again.

A clean colon, good food and regular exercise will make a huge difference in how you feel; and not just physically, but mentally. When you're "backed up" you can feel down and often depressed. I've treated clients who hadn't had a bowel movement for over two weeks. Two weeks! And when they receive a colonic, of course they're relieved to not be constipated, but they also feel happier.

Think about it from another perspective: When our body is full of old waste, full of nasty toxins, it has to work to try and keep that from making us even sicker than we might already be. And sometimes it isn't able to do so and in turn that waste becomes disease. But if our insides are cleaned out, then it lets our body focus on other areas. Our skin will start to look better, our eyes will be whiter and we'll have improved circulation. The kidneys, the gallbladder, the liver– they're all connected to the colon, and if it's backed up and not working, it affects them. If it's clean and working properly, then the other organs can do their jobs as well.

A colonic is so much more than just getting rid of the shit! A colonic could very well save your life.

4

But Is It Gonna Hurt?

No, not at all.

I'd like to introduce you to Sean, the graphic artist who designed the cover, inside of the book and was my consultant during the writing process. This is in his own words, which will be in italics, with my comments here and there.

Hi, Sean here, Karin thought it appropriate that I experience her various treatments, most specifically colonics, in order to better understand what she does. So for seven consecutive weeks I received a colonic.

It definitely doesn't hurt, but it is, shall we say, interesting to have a speculum inserted into the butt. All I had to do was take a few deep breaths and after a while you kind of forget it's even there.

When I arrived for the first session, Karin had me fill out a questionnaire that covered any symptoms I might be experiencing: constipation, fatigue and so on. It was very thorough and would allow her to address anything specific I might be dealing with.

Next, you empty the bladder and put on one of those hospital gowns. You know, with your backside there for everyone to see. Fortunately, it's only Karin and I! And for the record, this is the first time a client of mine has seen my nether regions. I can't recall any graphic design jobs that require one drop trough!

You lay face up on what looks like a massage table. Karin points to two very detailed illustrations on the wall and explains different areas of, and problems that can occur, within the colon. Then it's time. Roll over on your side, take a deep breath and help her gently insert the speculum into your bum. She uses organic coconut oil as the lubricant. Funny, how you can cook and "clean" with the same substance. Then, she attaches the intake and release tubes to the speculum and you roll back over on your back. Next, she places a cylindrical pillow under your knees, followed by a warm blanket to keep you comfy and relaxed. And I must say, after a few moments, it really is very relaxing.

I'd had a colonic about twenty years ago and remember it feeling rushed and definitely with frequent discomfort. The woman that administered it seemed to be going through the motions and didn't really care how effective it was as long as my check cleared.

That's the opposite with Karin, she's very hands-on and I

mean that literally. Now before you get gross thoughts in your head, let me explain. First, everything is very antiseptic, just like a doctor's office or hospital. Secondly, she gently massages your colon with her hands (from the outside), which not only helps the water to be effective with its cleaning of your colon, it allows Karin to know where things are clogged, where gas is hanging out, and just gives her an overall sense of what state your colon is in. Remember, she's the Shit Whisperer – a name that's well-deserved!

As the water fills the colon you start to feel full, like you have to go; but again it's not really uncomfortable, you just know it's time to release. And then it happens. To some, this may seem nasty as you watch your body's waste stream through a clear tube and out to the sewer system, just like your toilet. But to know you're getting rid of built-up waste and toxins, soon makes it something you look forward to as you get more and more treatments. There's a certain satisfaction knowing that you're becoming cleaner and cleaner with each release and subsequent treatment.

The session lasts about forty-five minutes. Each time you release, Karin can add a bit more water to get further into your colon. The first session really only does superficial cleaning, but I can say for fact, I immediately noticed a difference. Even while still cleaning and releasing, I felt a tingly sensation all over my body. Karin explained that because of the release of toxins. As we wrapped up the session, I used her restroom to get rid of everything else that was ready to release. I stood up to get dressed and noticed my eye sight was clearer. No, my eyesight didn't actually improve, but because I'd gotten rid of the waste and toxins, my eyes had an easier time doing their job.

My gut did feel a little funky right after the treatment, but that quickly turned into a feeling of emptiness. And I don't mean a lonely feeling, I mean a feeling of clean! It was invigorating!

When it comes to the first session, we're just getting started. I always recommend at least three sessions, so we can get the built-up waste loosened and flushed out. One is always beneficial, but typically only releases recent waste, not the old stuff — and that's what we're really going after. That's where the toxins are, plaque and very old, dark, muddy, black fecal matter. It might sound gross to some, but I think it's even grosser having it inside your body. Let's get it out!

My second treatment was the only one where I experienced a little bit of discomfort, which Karin assured me was normal. And it was hardly painful, I just felt overly full sooner than I had the previous week. And Karin is not one to be cruel, if you let her know or she senses you're feeling pressure or any discomfort, she immediately releases — and then that feeling is gone instantly.

I'd just finished my third treatment, told Karin goodbye and headed towards my car. I immediately noticed I felt lighter—like I'd lost weight. I returned and told Karin. She smiled and said we'd released between two and three pounds of waste during that session! That was just crazy to me. Crazy to think how full of shit more of us are. Literally and figuratively!

Nothing significant occurred during the fourth and fifth

sessions other than always feeling clean and empty afterward. Originally, we'd only planned for me to have six treatments. But during the sixth session we started to make some major progress and I had significant releases. I was honestly astonished about how much came out of my body. I felt the tingly sensation again and truly felt lighter once more. And another positive side effect of a colonic is a mood enhancer. You feel like you can take on the world. Your body isn't bogged down with all this old gunk and can actually do its job. It's such a wonderful feeling.

It was time for my seventh colonic and I figured there would be decent results, but since I had such a significant series of releases the previous week, I didn't expect anything amazing. Well, that'll teach me to be pessimistic! At first, it was like any other treatment, a little release here and there and then about thirty minutes in, the flood gates opened! Karin was like a proud mother watching her kid win the spelling bee. "This is why we did another treatment" she beamed. And there was another. I thought that was about it, but Karin said you have one more. All by her magical touch — and she was right!

Sean hit the jackpot with this seventh treatment. It just goes to show how much garbage is stuck inside our bodies. You didn't eat twenty years of food at once, you certainly can't expect that much waste to release right away. Your colon is an organ and a muscle and muscles get fatigued. We have to gently clean it, in short sessions, so it can begin to do its job more efficiently. That's why multiple sessions are important. Trying to go for one long session just doesn't work. The colon needs time to recover as well. Once a week is typically the best bet.

From Sean's first session until the seventh, I noticed several things. First, his skin glowed. He had dark circles under his eyes that were nearly gone. He looked healthier and seemed happier. And that means I've done my job.

> I can't emphasize enough how satisfying it is to get the waste out of your body. Anyone that knows me, knows I'm incredibly uncomfortable talking about "number two" but when you're able to truly clean your body and feel the amazing benefits that come from it, I'm okay with that. Especially if it might inspire others to improve their health.
>
> It's funny, but when you have a good, long release, Karin actually gets excited. She truly gains satisfaction from getting the shit out. I mean it in the way that she's a healer and helper and someone who cares. She wants everyone to be okay talking about it. Perhaps not at dinner or at a holiday gathering, but in general, shit isn't a dirty word. Hey, that's a good title for a book!
>
> Since my treatments, I've noticed less bloating after I eat, less discomfort, more mental clarity and go figure, my pants don't feel quite as tight. I'm a supporter of taking care of your gut and it'll take care of you. I don't always eat as healthy as I should, most of us don't, but I do try my best—and I most definitely plan on keeping up with the colonics.
>
> In my lay opinion, getting regular colonics could literally add years to your life.

I couldn't agree more, Sean.

5

They Still Wanted to Poison Me

First-hand experience from a cancer survivor.

I'd like to introduce one of my clients, Elba Rojas. Elba is a breast cancer and chemotherapy survivor. This is her story in her own words.

Hello, I'm Elba. I'm fifty-six years old. For the past thirty years I worked as a project manager for an interpreting & translating agency. The job was very stressful. A lot of office politics and drama that I had to deal with on a daily basis. After about twenty years on the job, I started getting sick. I had stomach problems and didn't feel like myself. This went on for about ten years before I discovered what was wrong.

This last year I went in for a mammogram. Afterwards, they told me I had to come back and be re-tested. That's something no one wants to hear, but I had to accept it. After my second mammogram, they took me aside and said I had two tumors in my right breast. One was two centimeters and the other was one centimeter in diameter. I was in shock—I couldn't believe it. It doesn't run in my family. How could this be true? But it was.

The doctors felt it was brought on by unhealthy eating and stress. I knew they were right. They scheduled my surgery within two weeks from my diagnosis.

I was willing to have a complete mastectomy; I didn't care. I just wanted it out of my body. The surgeon told me that wasn't necessary, that she does this all the time. The tumors were close together and it would be a simple task to remove them. They used a contrast dye in my breast to check if the cancer had spread, and it had. One nearby lymph node was affected. They removed both tumors, the lymph node and left a safety margin in the vicinity of where the tumors were, just to be safe. I was concerned it may have spread to other lymph nodes, but they assured me it hadn't.

After my surgery, I was essentially cancer free, but the doctors first wanted me to receive radiation and then they said I should also have chemotherapy treatments.

It was about a month later that I started Docetaxel-cisplatin*, which is very aggressive and very expensive chemotherapy combination. Fortunately my insurance covered it.

Karin here: in my experience, doctors will often prescribe what's "in stock," what's "profitable" and what provides an off-the-record commission or kickback, if you will, from the pharmaceutical company.

NOT what's necessarily best for the patient. Or even necessary at all. I've said it before — not all doctors are bad or greedy, but many of them are. Some provide wonderful, thoughtful care and put the patient's health and wellness ahead of anything else, including money. Some start out good and eventually get sucked into the money-machine by prescribing expensive drugs that insurance companies are often forced to cover. It's sad, but very, very true.

> My chemo treatments were in four cycles, three weeks apart. The day after the treatment, I was a mess. Terribly constipated with all the poison they were pumping into my body. It was horrible. For three days after each chemo session, I had to give myself injections to stimulate the growth of bone marrow; which was to fight off infections and produce more white blood cells. That was so painful. I could barely walk afterward. That entire week was hell.
>
> The second week after chemo I would start to feel a little better, except for the constipation. That was so uncomfortable. Nothing I ate would pass. By the third week, I would finally be feeling much, much better only to have to do it all over again.
>
> After I completed the chemo, I had a three week break and then started radiation. Five days a week, for four weeks, I received radiation treatments. It looked like I had a bad sunburn which caused my skin to peel. I was so fatigued. I just sat around, took frequent naps and couldn't do much of anything.
>
> I'd taken a medical leave from my job when the chemo began and I eventually resigned. I couldn't go back to that level of stress. Not after what I've been through. Thank goodness I qualified for disability.

Once I completed my radiation, I asked the doctors what was next. They told me to start living a normal life; I was cancer free. I was happy to hear I didn't have cancer any longer, but it didn't seem right to go back to my normal life. My body had been flooded with poison and burned with radiation. There had to be more to it than that. I started doing research.

First, I read about juicing. Healthy, clean juices that will help flush away the toxins left over from the treatments. I was about to begin that detox, when I discovered Karin and Pure Center. I'd heard about colonics, but had never had one. I knew nothing about it and had no idea what to expect, but I wanted to do the right thing.

Karin was able to take me right away. I was scared at first. But she was kind, compassionate and made me feel comfortable. After the first colonic, I found my constipation was gone. In fact, I found myself going to the bathroom all the time! I was happy that the bad stuff was coming out of me, but in doing so, it also made me fatigued once again. All that toxin being released, takes its toll on your body. But it was a step in the right direction and I was totally okay with that.

The second and third colonic sessions were definitely uncomfortable. As Karin would fill my colon with water, I would feel pressure. She would immediately release. My body was so full of toxins and built-up waste that was finally coming out; it was just lot for my body to handle.

Finally, after a few more treatments, I really started to feel a whole lot better. When I first saw Karin, my fingernails were nearly black, had cracks and were very fragile. Now, they are almost completely clear and firm. My hair has grown back, my eyes are whiter and my skin is clear.

Since I've been receiving weekly colonics, I'm slowly getting back to my normal self. At first, I could barely eat, mostly soups, as it would go right through me. I was weak and my emotions were raw. I'm very lucky to have a supportive husband and family that stuck by me through this very difficult time. Thank God for them.

I still get a little weak and tired after a colonic, but my recovery is much faster and each time, I feel little a bit better, stronger and happier. Now, I'm starting to prepare organic meals and attempting to get my family to go along with a healthier lifestyle. My husband is stubborn, but that's okay. I'll keep working on him. I do feel that if I'd eaten healthier early on I might not have gotten cancer — who knows.

I'm not a doctor and I'm not an expert when it comes to cancer treatment, but in my opinion, I did not need chemo or radiation. I think Karin would agree. I'm not recovering from my cancer surgery, that didn't take very long at all. But nine months later, I am still recovering from and feeling the effects of, poisoning and radiating my body. Plus, I had to experience painful injections to replenish the lost bone marrow caused by the chemotherapy. That doesn't make much sense, if you ask me. Shame on the doctors who do this for profit and don't have the patient's best interest in mind.

But something good did come out of all of this. I'm living a much healthier lifestyle, I'm happier, I feel at peace and I can call this amazing, kind and caring person, Karin, a friend. God bless you.

6

My Husband & I Could Not Get Pregnant

But not for lack of trying! Well, my husband couldn't get pregnant no matter what, but we tried for many years to get me pregnant and it just wouldn't happen.

It was about two years before we were married that we decided we wanted to start a family. First step was to make sure everything was good from the health aspect. We went to the doctor and sure enough my soon-to-be husband's sperm count was good, my eggs were good; we were ready to make a baby!

First year: Nothing. Second year: Same. Our doctor suggested insemination. They took my husband's sperm, cleaned it and injected it directly into me during my ovulation. Meanwhile, I was taking a hormone supplement to allegedly make me more receptive to getting pregnant. The process took about six weeks. First I'd take the hormones, they'd inseminate me precisely when my ovulation cycle was perfect. Then we'd wait. I'd call the doctor. Bad news; Not pregnant. We did this three more times over the course of the year only to be disappointed each time.

During the last insemination treatment, I told the doctor that it wasn't going to work; that I wasn't ovulating. She said according to all the tests, you are. I insisted that I wasn't, I knew my body and I didn't feel it. I knew that it was a waste of time and certainly a waste of money. And I was right!

To make matters worse, those hormones made me look like shit, feel like shit and mixed with the frustration of not getting pregnant, it was not a happy time. The doctor kept assuring us we were both healthy and just to be patient. At this point sex wasn't enjoyable, it had become work. It wasn't something either of us looked forward to, we just did it out of obligation.

At this point sex wasn't enjoyable, it had become work.

I quickly learned that for the average person, getting pregnant isn't all that easy, especially if you're a little older and at this time, I was about thirty-one. Of course, then I'd get a call from a friend who said, "I got pregnant accidentally!" I didn't want to hear it. Certainly I was happy for her, but I had no interest in attending baby showers or any sort of celebration as it was a reminder that I couldn't get pregnant. And this happened more than once. All these women getting pregnant — except me!

Both my husband and I lived healthy lives, no drugs, took care of ourselves, so we really thought getting pregnant would be easy. We couldn't have been more wrong, but were more than willing to do whatever it took for it to work. If someone had said to stand on my head, I would've done it. We were determined!

My doctor suggested IVF (In Vitro Fertilization: Whereby the women's egg is fertilized by sperm in a test tube or elsewhere outside the body). We decided we'd try it, but not here in the U.S. because it's quite expensive. I think somewhere around $50,000 at the time. But first, I needed to stop the hormone treatments and clean my body of everything, including the stress of trying and failing at getting pregnant.

The hormones made me constipated, which is something a person who gives (and receives) colonics is not used to. But if we were going to be successful with the IVF treatment, I wanted my body to be as clean as possible. I began a treatment of over twenty colonics. First, once a day for the first six; then every other day and the last series were every three days. I ate clean, I did everything I could to be as healthy as possible, I even fasted a few times. I did a liver flush with lemon and olive oil to remove toxins; as well as coffee enemas to help stimulate the production of bile which also helps flush the body.

I began to feel vibrant, energized. I truly felt amazing after my cleanse. My husband and I also saw the return of the desire for intimacy, which leads of course to sex. Sex we wanted to have, not sex we had to have! So much more enjoyable!

> **My husband and I also saw the return of the desire for intimacy, which leads of course to sex.**

My doctor did suggest I take an estrogen hormone just to get everything in balance since we still wanted to get pregnant. She told me to take them for about ten days. If I get my period, continue. If I don't, then stop. I figured that would be okay.

Now it was time to get started with the IVF, but I wasn't doing that here, I was going to travel to Israel. Plus, I was going to see my brother because he and his wife just had a baby! Can you believe it?

My husband scheduled appointments with the top doctors in Israel. We wanted to get a second opinion on my health and readiness for getting pregnant before we moved forward with the IVF treatment. The plan was for the Israeli doctor to prescribe the medications; I would pick them up in Israel and bring them back with me to the U.S. for the actual procedure.

Once I got to Israel, I was feeling great. In a good mood, really ready to relax and enjoy myself. I went to the bris for my brother's son (The Jewish circumcision ceremony). We had some wine, some cocktails, nothing crazy, but I definitely relaxed and decompressed.

When I saw the doctor, he gave me an ultrasound and told me I was ovulating. I said, "That's fantastic, but my husband's not here!" He agreed that I was healthy and prescribed the IVF.

Over the course of the next week I began to feel fatigued. I wasn't sure why, but figured it was because of what I'd been through, plus traveling. I went to the pharmacy to order the IVF prescription. The pharmacist asked if I was sure I wanted this, because it cost $3,000 and is not refundable. I assured him I did, so he placed the order and said to return the next day to pick it up.

I had gone to the shopping mall with my sister and despite knowing I wasn't pregnant and being a little tired, I was happy. I was having a nice time. Since I was taking the estrogen supplement, if I got my period, then I would continue, but if not, I had to stop. So I picked up a pregnancy test, peed on the stick as you do and when it showed two lines, I thought I must've grabbed an ovulation test by mistake. I went back and bought another pregnancy test. I peed again and got the same result — pregnant! I showed it to my sister and she assured me it was both a pregnancy test and it was saying I was pregnant.

Off to another doctor I went. He drew some blood and said he'd give me the results shortly. The next day he called my mother to tell her congratulations that I was two months pregnant! I couldn't believe it! Had my other doctor, the one that gave me the ultrasound and prescribed the IVF, given me a blood test, I would've saved the cost of the expensive drugs I now no longer needed.

I had to laugh. Yeah, we'd just spent $3,000 on drugs we don't need, but I'm pregnant! Yay! My mom and entire family were elated I was finally with child! Now I had to let my husband know.

I called him and said, "I have good news and really good news." I told him I just picked up the IVF drugs. He said, "Great, we'll get started once you return. What's the other good news?" I smiled, "I'm two months pregnant!" He couldn't believe either, but was equally as excited.

It had taken us nearly three years and we ended up having a natural pregnancy. All because the pressure of trying to get pregnant was no longer there and my body was clean.

Seven months later, our beautiful baby daughter was born. We've since joked with her that she was a very expensive child! But as they say, things happen for a reason and we wouldn't want it any other way,

    Since my experience I have helped many women who could not get pregnant otherwise, finally succeed with colonic treatments. I get great pleasure when I get the call that they've gotten pregnant. It makes what I do all the more worthwhile.

7

A Spiritual Cleanse

I'd like to introduce you to another one of my clients, Lee Ann Smith. Lee has been through a great deal in her life and this is her experience.

> I've been receiving colonics for more than twenty years. It started after I was diagnosed with IBS (Irritable Bowel Syndrome) in the '90s. I've been to many different colonic therapists and Karin is hands down, the best, the most gentle, kindest, funniest, sweetest — she really makes getting the shit out a pleasant experience! She's highly educated and she cares about her clients. That's so important to me, to receive treatment from someone that treats me with dignity and respect, and isn't just in it for the money. She's the utmost professional, but always with a personal, human touch. I can't say enough about her!

I have other medical issues that I'm dealing with and have had to have surgeries. So it's important that prior to the surgery, treatment, procedure or whatever it may be, that my colon is clean. I also have trouble digesting and receiving nutrients from food, so the colonics help to keep things in check. Your health starts with the gut. I've known that for a very a long time.

Years ago when I first began receiving colonics, and this is before I'd met Karin, there was a lot of negativity surrounding this sort of treatment. Doctors would say that colonics remove good bacteria. Well, if we ate properly we wouldn't need to worry, but we don't; and our food source in the U.S. is so poor, no wonder people aren't healthy. It's really sad. If you take probiotics and eat healthy, you'll be doing your body a favor. Sure, you'll still need a colonic now and again, but not as often if you're taking care of yourself. In fact, back then a lot of people would use colonics to lose weight. That's not what a colonic does, it helps remove your body's waste, not fat. The upside, having a clean colon can help you naturally lose weight because your body is more efficient, but you still need to take care of yourself, regardless.

Another issue is medications. Because of my health issues, I have to take a variety of medications and they mess with the gut, big time. At one point I hadn't had a bowel movement in nearly thirty days, which is quite painful. My regular colonic therapist, at the time, wasn't available, so I had to find someone else. I was nervous, because not only are you put into a very vulnerable scenario, it can also be very uncomfortable and if the therapist isn't gentle, the pain can be unbearable. That's when I found Karin and after my first treatment, I said, "Where have you been all my life?!"

I wish my health issues were the worst of my problems, but unfortunately not. My son was killed while serving in Afghanistan. It's been just over eight years now, but still feels like yesterday. The stress from losing your child is something I wouldn't wish upon anyone. This literally affects your well being, both mentally and physically. My doctors felt that this stress actually lead to new health problems. Your body can only take so much before it reacts. Having been through what I've experienced has taught me how to deal with and manage stress. This is also why I've created and support many charities that help both discharged military and their families never feel forgotten or that they aren't loved.

Forgetting health issues for the moment, stress itself can be the cause of your colon to acting up. It can cause constipation and a whole lot of other issues. But mix that with my health issues and I was practically a basket case! And you wouldn't tie a colonic to mental health, but amazingly so, they are one in the same. After receiving my numerous treatments from Karin, I felt a weight had been lifted off my chest. When you release the toxins and waste from your body, you are often unknowingly letting go of the past. Letting go of stress, letting go of what's metaphorically eating you up inside. It's truly a spiritual cleanse.

I completely agree with Lee on that one. My job is to

administer a colonic and make sure you receive the best possible treatment I can provide. But it's also a very intimate procedure. You get to know your clients and they feel comfortable talking with you. I've had clients tell me they've been in therapy for years with little result, but after receiving colonics they not only feel better physically, but emotionally. Perhaps there's a higher power involved, but I truly believe that when you get rid of old, built-up waste from years ago, you're also getting rid of old, built- up emotions as well. Our body is a complex mechanism with all things tied together in one way or another and emotions are a huge part of that. Just like Lee said, stress can cause constipation; that's emotions affecting our insides.

When you release toxins it affects the brain chemistry. You can suddenly feel emotional and not know why. Getting rid of toxins makes you feel better. You feel better, you're happier. Toxins affect us in so many ways. When we experience brain fog or feel sluggish, it's because of toxins. Our body can't be its efficient self with essentially poison inside of us. You get rid of the poison, you get rid of the problems.

There is also muscle memory. The tissues within our muscles have very good memories. And it's not just playing sports or repeating a complex task with ease, it's everything within us. Before my recent health issues, I would rarely get sick, except every year on my birthday. I never understood why. Finally, I was talking with my mother about it and she told me that when I was born, I was sick and had to stay in the hospital for a time afterward. Now that I was aware of this and did a little research, no longer was I sick on my birthday. Muscle memory had literally made me sick once a year because that's how I was when I was born and each year on my birthday it returned.

In order for us to heal, no matter what it is, we not only need to rid ourselves of waste, but of negative emotions and stress. I can't emphasize enough how our mind and body work together. When we're clean on the inside, we'll look and feel good on the outside. When those toxins aren't weighing you down, your body can work properly which affects your emotional well being. Something as simple as gas or feeling bloated can make you cranky; that's your body affecting your emotions. But when the gas is gone, so is the cranky feeling. Or let's say you're constipated and you realize that you've had a recent change in your life that's caused you stress. If you'll properly deal with the stress, which could mean seeing a therapist or just talking it out with a loved one or close friend—instead of taking a stimulant-based laxative, your constipation will begin to subside. In the process, go see Karin for a colonic, she'll help you not only release all that built-up waste, she'll help you feel better at the same time. I call that a win- win!

8

The Scoop on Poop

Some might consider it a necessary evil, while others actually find it satisfying. No matter how you might feel about it, shit happens. It's part of the digestive process; one of our body's many functions — and there's a great deal to learn and understand about this, rather amazing, process.

What exactly is poop?

It mostly consists of undigested foods, proteins, bacteria, salts and other substances that are produced and then released by our intestines. Although no one poop is created equal, the size, shape, and smell of one's poop indicates a healthy or not-so-healthy individual.

What's considered a normal poop?

There are many components that make up your poop and each one can be assessed to determine how healthy your poop might or might not be.

Color

Brown. Which is no surprise to most anyone. Bilirubin, a pigment compound formed from the breakdown of red blood cells within the body, is what gives our poop the oh-so-familiar brown hue.

Shape

A log-like shape is how a healthy poop should come out due to it's formation within your intestines. But there are a whole variety of different shapes that poop can take on. When your poop doesn't take on the log-like shape, that's when it's trying to tell you something might be wrong.

Consistency

Somewhere between firm and soft is fairly normal. If it goes towards one extreme or the other, then there might be some digestion or other issues.

Time on the pot

We've all shared a laugh when someone has taken too long in the bathroom, "They must be pooping!" But a healthy poop should be easy to release and only take about a minute to push out. That being said, many people do spend a bit more time on the pot than others, so it's safe to say a poop shouldn't take much more than ten to fifteen minutes. Besides, you don't want your butt to fall asleep, right?

How often do you go?

It's a known fact that most people poop around the same time everyday. Some, first thing in the morning; others, right after a meal. And some might leave it until the end of the day. Someone with healthy digestion will poop from as much as three times a day, to every other day. Any less could mean constipation and a need for more water to keep things flowing.

Size and Shape Matter

There are essentially seven categories of poop based upon size and consistency.

1. *Marbles*

Appearance: Hard & separate little clumps that look like nuts or marbles and are often hard to pass. Cause: These little guys usually mean you're constipated.

2. *Caterpillar*

Appearance: Log-shaped, but a little funky-looking. Cause: Another sign or form of constipation.

3. *Hot Dogs*

Appearance: Log-shaped with a few cracks on the outside. Cause: This is the ideal poop, especially if it's moderately firm and easy to pass.

4. *Snakes*

Appearance: Smooth and snake like Cause: This is also considered normal and should happen every few days.

5. *Amoebas*

Appearance: These guys are small like the marbles, but are soft and easier to pass. Cause: This means you're lacking fiber.

6. *Soft Serve*

Appearance: Fluffy and mushy, with rough edges. Cause: This very soft consistency could be a sign of mild diarrhea.

7. Jackson Pollack (the abstract artist)

Appearance: Entirely liquid with no solid matter. Cause: This means you've got the runs or diarrhea. Your stool moved through your bowels very quickly and didn't form into a healthy poop.

Let's Talk About Color

Much like size and shape, the color of your poop can also help us know what's going on inside our bodies. Various shades of brown are considered normal, and believe it or not, according to the Mayo Clinic, a slight hint of green is just fine too. But if your poop is taking on colors of the rainbow, it's time to give it some consideration.

Black

If you've had licorice, iron supplements, or medications like Pepto-Bismal, that could cause your stool to be black. Black poop can also be an indication of bleeding in the upper GI tract. Logic would say it would appear to be red in this instance, but since it takes a bit to travel down, it's older and darker.

Green

Hints of green are perfectly normal. But if it's more green than brown, or completely green, it means you've either added a great deal green foods like spinach to your diet, or your stool is passing through you too quickly.

Pale, White or Clay Colored

If your poop is a very light shade, it might mean you're lacking bile. Bile comes from your liver and gallbladder and aides in digestion. If you're producing an almost white stool, it means your bile duct might be blocked.

It could also be a side-effect for medications like an anti-diarrhea. If it continues, consult your doctor.

Red

Red poop can obviously mean bleeding, from hemorrhoids or bleeding in the lower intestine, but if your stool is red occasionally, there's usually no worry; unless it continues.

Foods like beets, cranberries, red gelatin and tomato juice can also turn your poop red.

Yellow

Greasy, stink, yellow poop is usually a sign of too much fat. This could also be because of celiac disease, where your body isn't absorbing enough nutrients.

Ooo, Ooo, That Smell!

Nobody's poop smells particularly great; even if, for some bizarre unexplainable reason, you think it does, trust me, no one else does! But if you've noticed that yours is even more fragrant than normal, it might be a sign that something's going on in your body.

There are 10 trillion microorganisms living in the human GI tract — yes trillion! The odor of your poop is created by the gases that are produced in the intestine when non-absorbable carbs (fiber) become fermented.

If your poop smells kind of funky for a day or two, no big deal—it's probably something you ate. But if the funk isn't going away, then it's worth talking to your doctor; especially if the consistency of your poop has changed too. This could be a sign of any number of issues, from a food allergy/intolerance, irritable bowel syndrome (IBS), a nutrient malabsorption issue, bleeding somewhere in the digestive tract, or an infection.

What happens if my poop is floating?

It's not a toy boat, don't play with it! It just means that the stool is less dense than the others that sink. One reason can be from an increased amount of gas or water. Another may be malabsorption, which would present other issues such as constipation.

What if I'm Constipated?

Try and avoid taking a laxative. There are a variety reasons, including stress, that can cause constipation. One of the best and healthiest ways to relieve that clogged-up feeling is a colonic. Water is used to clean the colon, not a stimulant; the latter of which can be quite unpleasant and not nearly as effective. Once you've had a colonic or series of them, now it's time to add more high-fiber foods to your diet, drink lots of healthy fluids, stay active and manage your stress to avoid becoming constipated again.

When Should I See My Doctor?

A little abnormal pooping happens to all of us and you shouldn't worry. But when the abnormality continues for a few days or longer, then you should talk to your doctor. Pay attention to your poop! It might seem odd at first, but before you flush, take a look. Is there any blood or is your stool red, but you haven't had any of the foods to cause this? Is the color pale or solid green? Time to see the doctor before things get worse.

Like I've mentioned so many times in this book, maintain a healthy lifestyle and management of stress — your poop will be a semi-firm log and a beautiful shade of brown!

9

Health, Wellness, And Tasty Tidbits

I've said numerous times throughout this book that we need to take care of our insides. Besides a healthy diet, and I've included some of my favorite and quite tasty recipes at the end of this chapter for you, but we must also help our gut work properly with a few things that we can't necessarily get entirely from the food we eat.

Probiotics

Probiotics are live bacteria and yeasts that are good for you, especially your digestive system. They are also a bit of a mystery as to exactly how they work, because we usually think of these as germs that cause diseases. But your body is full of bacteria, both good and bad. Probiotics are often called "good" or "helpful" bacteria because they help keep your gut healthy. You can find probiotics in supplements and some foods, like yogurt. Doctors often suggest them to help with digestive problems. When you lose "good" bacteria in your body, for example after you take antibiotics, probiotics can help replace them. They can help balance your "good" and "bad" bacteria to keep your body working the way it should.

Many types of bacteria are classified as probiotics. They all have different benefits, but most come from three groups: Lactobacillus, Bifidobacterium, and Saccharomyces.

Lactobacillus. This may be the most common probiotic. It's the one you'll find in yogurt and other fermented foods. Different strains can help with diarrhea and may help people who can't digest lactose, the sugar in milk.

Bifidobacterium. You can find it in some dairy products. It may help ease the symptoms of irritable bowel syndrome (IBS) and some other conditions.

Saccharomyces boulardii is a yeast found in probiotics. It appears to help fight diarrhea and other digestive problems. Among other things, probiotics help send food through your gut by affecting nerves that control gut movement. They can help with Irritable Bowel Syndrome (IBS), Inflammatory Bowel Disease (IBD), and Infectious Diarrhea (caused by viruses, bacteria, or parasites). Probiotics can also help with skin conditions, like eczema, urinary and vaginal health, preventing allergies and colds, and oral health.

Ask your doctor about which might best help you.

Vitamin D

Vitamin D is a fat-soluble vitamin that is naturally present in very few foods, added to others, and available as a dietary supplement. It is also produced endogenously when ultraviolet rays from sunlight strike the skin and trigger vitamin D synthesis.

Without sufficient vitamin D, bones can become thin, brittle, or misshapen. Vitamin D sufficiency prevents rickets in children and osteomalacia in adults. Together with calcium, vitamin D also helps protect older adults from osteoporosis. Vitamin D has other roles in the body, including modulation of cell growth, neuromuscular and immune function, and reduction of inflammation. However, many of us are walking around with Vitamin D deficiencies and don't even know it. A simple blood test can determine if you are, and then your doctor can prescribe a higher dose than you can get over the counter if you are in fact lacking enough Vitamin D.

Vitamin B12

Vitamin B12 is a nutrient that helps keep the body's nerve and blood cells healthy and helps make DNA, the genetic material in all our cells. Vitamin B12 also helps prevent megaloblastic anemia which makes people tired and weak.

A great deal of vegetarians and vegans are severely lacking B12, because it is found naturally in a wide variety of animal foods, but not in plant-based foods unless they are fortified. Whether or not you eat or animal products, it's important that your body has proper amount of B12, which means taking a good-quality supplement. Beef liver and clams, are the best sources of vitamin B12. Fish, meat, poultry, eggs, milk, and other dairy products, also contain vitamin B12.

> **Whether or not you eat or animal products, it's important that your body has proper amount of B12**

Some breakfast cereals, nutritional yeasts and other food

products are fortified with vitamin B12. To find out if vitamin B12 has been added to a food product, check the product labels.

The Wonder Tonic: Celery Juice!

There are many proven health benefits of drinking celery juice. Celery has powerful anti-inflammatory effects, due to the phytosterol (a group of naturally occurring compounds found in plant cell membranes) and unidentified polar substances. These anti-inflammatory properties can help with acid reflux, bloating, IBS, constipation, acne, eczema, and other inflammation issues in the body. Celery juice is very high in vitamin K which promotes general bone and heart health, and high in vitamin C, which is critical for your immune system.

Because of celery's diuretic properties (high water content) and the fact that it contains magnesium, phthalides (which relaxes the tissues of the artery walls to increase blood flow) and potassium — celery may actually help those with high blood pressure. And its bioactive flavonoids help to fight and prevent cancer cells. Can't get much more wonderful than that!

Magnesium

Magnesium is the fourth most abundant mineral in the human body and plays several important roles in the health of your body and brain. Magnesium is a mineral found in the earth, sea, plants, animals and humans. About 60% of the magnesium in your body is found in bone, while the rest is in muscles, soft tissues and fluids, including blood. In fact, every cell in your body contains it and needs it to function.

Simply put, Magnesium helps convert food into energy; helps

create new proteins from amino acids; helps create and repair DNA and RNA; is part of the contraction and relaxation of muscles; and helps regulate neurotransmitters, which send messages throughout your brain and nervous system.

Most grocery stores, drug stores and health food stores offer over-the-counter Magnesium supplements as well as online sources like Amazon. As always, consult your doctor as to what's best for you.

Now that you've learned how to supplement your healthy diet, I bet you're hungry. Let's make some tasty dishes that are also good for you!

Moroccan Salmon

Ingredients:

6 Salmon Filets (4-6oz)
2 Tomatoes, diced
1 14oz Can Chickpeas or Garbanzo Beans, drained
5 Garlic Cloves, peeled, crushed and roughly chopped
2 Jalapeños, stems and seeds removed; diced
1 Carrot, diced
1 Bunch Cilantro, chopped
1 Lemon, sliced into rounds
I Tablespoon Olive Oil
1/2 Teaspoon Cumin
1/2 Teaspoon Red Sweet Paprika
1/2 Teaspoon Kosher Salt, plus more to taste
1 Cup Water, more as needed

Method:

Put a large, deep skillet with a tight-fitting lid, over medium heat. Once hot, add the olive oil, allow it to begin to thin out, then add the tomatoes, jalapeños, carrots, chickpeas and sweat for 2-3 minutes. Add garlic and cook for no more than 30 seconds to prevent it from burning. Add the spices, stir to combine and add about a tablespoon or two of water to open it up and just cover the vegetables.

Evenly space the salmon filets atop the vegetables, cover with lemon slices and spread with the cilantro. Reduce the heat to low, cover and simmer for approximately 45 minutes. Periodically check, adding water if necessary. Salmon should be cooked until it reaches an internal temperature of 145 F (63 degrees C). Check for seasoning, add salt if desired.

Serve with veggies and pan drippings. Optional sides: quinoa or brown rice and challah bread.

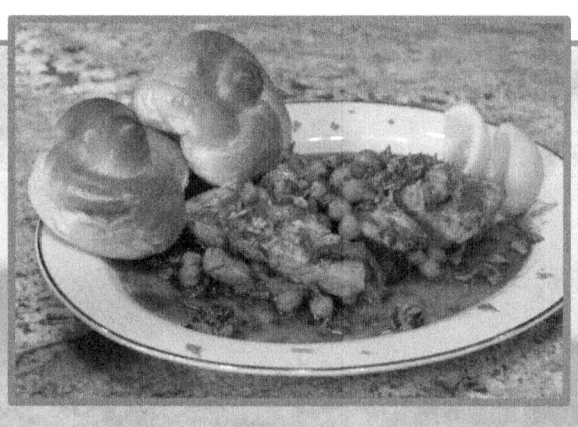

HUMMUS

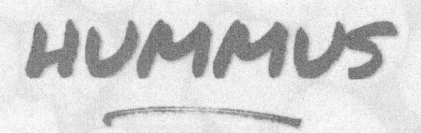

Ingredients:
- 1 15oz can Chickpeas (also known as Garbanzo Beans), rinsed and drained. Reserve a tablespoon's worth for garnish.
- 1/4 cup lemon juice (from 1 1/2 to 2 lemons), more to taste
- 2-3 medium garlic cloves
- 1/2 teaspoon fine Kosher salt, to taste
- 1/2 cup tahini
- 1/2 tablespoons ice water, more as needed
- 1 teaspoon ground cumin
- 1 tablespoon extra-virgin olive oil, plus more for garnish
- Chopped Italian parsley for garnish
- Paprika for garnish

Method: Place all of your ingredients in a food processor and blend until smooth, add more water if needed, a little a time, until you get a delightful creamy texture. Serve with some whole chickpeas, a drizzle of Olive Oil and dusting of paprika or experiment with other garnishes to your liking.

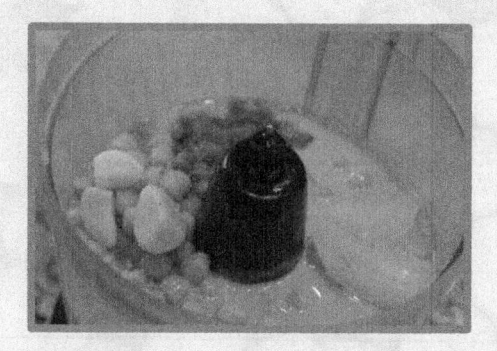

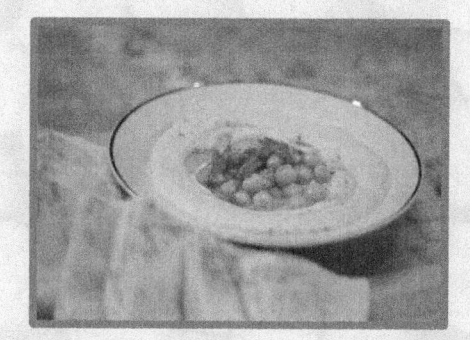

10

Other Forms of Detox

Besides colonics, there are many other forms of detox to put you on the path to health and wellness. Our muscles and our skin, both hold toxins. Increasing and stimulating circulation is key to keeping things flowing within our bodies.

Here are just a few of other treatments I offer my clients in conjunction with colonics or as stand-alone detox treatments.

Massage

Most think of a massage only for pleasure. Certainly they are enjoyable and relaxing, but they also are detox. By stimulating the skin and muscles, toxins are released and eliminated from the body.

Iridology Retina Scan

A small device is placed over each eye and records patterns, colors and other characteristics which can determine a patient's systemic health.

After analysis, this allows our technician to recommend services to improve one's health. This can also provide information on potential health risks before they become serious, allowing our client to see their doctor for appropriate testing.

Ear Coning

This ancient detox and healing practice uses a 100% beeswax-dipped muslin cone to gently help balance ear conditions. Each session gently draw debris out of the ear canal, often dramatically improving one's hearing.

Cupping

Another ancient form of alternative medicine and detox in which a therapist puts special cups on your skin for a few minutes to create suction. It helps with pain, inflammation, blood flow, relaxation and well-being, and as a type of deep-tissue massage.

FAR Infrared Sauna

An excellent tool to aid in cleansing, detoxing and flushing toxicity from your body. It has been said to aid in weight loss and be especially beneficial for the elimination of heavy metals. FAR uses infrared light to heat you up instead of using conduction (through the hot wood) or through convection (heated air or steam.) Infrared light is part of the sun's invisible spectrum. FAR Infrared Sauna uses the far part of the safe infrared spectrum. Infrared light is the exact opposite end of the light spectrum and is associated with many positive and healthful effects.

Iconic Foot Bath

This relaxes, cleanses, balances and enhances the bioenergy of the body. The feet are a channel or conduit through which the body cleanses itself of toxic wastes and heavy metals that build up in the blood. With the Ionic Foot Bath you can assist your system in eliminating toxins, yeast and unwanted debris as the process results in the correct frequency required for the cells to return to a healthy state, because the blood no longer has impurities that weigh the cells down. They become clear and fully charged, resulting in a positive attitude, more energy and enables the body to heal itself.

Do some research to see if your colonic therapist also offers treatments such as these, or seek out someone that does. You won't be disappointed!

Epilogue: Marching Orders!

Unless you're doing a book report on my book, the fact that you've gotten to the end tells me you're serious about your health and wellness.

Now you have the knowledge, information, a few interesting stories, and a couple tasty recipes to try, that should inspire you to take the next steps to improving your health. Don't wait until the first of the year, no one keeps their New Year's Resolutions that I've ever met, and don't even wait until tomorrow. Take a positive step today! Right now. Even if it's just doing a little research, that's a good beginning. I'll be watching you! Okay, not really, that would be impossible and kind of creepy. But let me be your motivation. You've got your marching orders, now follow them and never look back. That's the old you. The new you is a health & wellness rock star. I'm already very proud of you! And you should be proud of yourself.

Your body is your temple and you're stuck with it for the rest of your life. Treat it with kindness, love and respect — and in turn , it will give you an enjoyable, happy and productive life.

Aren't you worth it? I know you are.

All my love,

Karin

Afterword

Genita M. Mason H.H.P., N.C., F.E.

Colon Hydrotherapy – For Some The Secret To Longevity & Energy To Others A Life Saving Procedure

Are You Really Dumping Your Garbage Dump When You Pooh?

It is a well-known fact that oxidative stress, which is simply more harmful toxic substances going into a person than the body can efficiently metabolize and remove, is the number one cause of all disease except that which may be genetic but oxidative stress will certainly expedite its progression, leaving the person much less time to find and exercise a solution. Oxidative stress is the beginning of the end if no well-organized and professionally assisted intervention is sought once symptoms begin. Symptoms tell you you're doing something wrong and the professional healthcare provider will not only help you identify what you're doing wrong, but they will help you detoxify your body and help you rebuild a healthy one.

When it comes to oxidative stress being the ground zero for all disease, unfortunately that 35 feet of gut from the tip of one's tongue to the poop shoot is a literal landfill in many people and becomes toxic from the rotting decomposition of undigested food and environmental and dietary toxins which accumulate in the colon and begin releasing into the blood system more and more biotoxins daily which recirculate poisons throughout the system including every organ. To make matters worse, these toxins begin to create their own toxins called lipopolysaccharides (LPS) – endotoxins. People suffering this condition today are diagnosed in the alternative medicine community as those with biotoxin illness – and this group of patients are now the lion's share of patients due to the mass adulteration and processing of food, environmental toxic assaults, and poor judgement when it comes to drugs and alcohol.

Gut health is so vital to overall health and so key to the cause of disease and metabolic syndromes that today it is the cornerstone focus of all healthcare practitioners worthy of consideration. For the last 20 years I have always run functional gut health Organic Acids Tests on all of my patients which tests for bacteria, fungus, yeast, inflammation, fat & blood in the stool and when in the late 90's possibly one in ten would have a dysbiosis or condition that required treatment, honestly I can't remember the last time I saw results that didn't have multiple serious issues. Air, water, lifestyle (which includes bad diets and lack of exercise), psychiatric and other prescription drugs (antibiotics being worse on gut health) and recreational drugs and stress all contribute to the estimated 9 out of 10 people suffering gut health issues and the diseases a toxin manufacturing plant a gut full of poisons stuck to its lining will cause. The gut is not a one-way out organ like most people believe. Even if you don't have leaky gut syndrome, toxins in your gut enter the blood system via the mesenteric arteries that wrap around it meant to absorb the short chain fatty acids from the fermentation of resistant starches and inulins in the colon the body uses for health oriented biological processes. **Leaky gut or "intestinal permeability"** only refers to particles larger than nature intended leaking from the gut. However, toxins are of molecular size and can be much, much smaller than fatty acids!

Being that I am the creator of an award-winning biological medicine medical model and the owner and Medical Director of the clinic that executes it, my clinic is at the cutting edge of the both ancient and modern sciences that support the best of biological medicine. To say the least, our success attracts the best of the best worldwide, and over the 20 years I've been in practice I must say I have been both blessed and spoiled with the world class practitioners in all the treatments that we offer in synergistic treatment packages that include ozone blood purification, medical hydrogen, nutritional and brain restorative IVs, Pulse Electromagnetic Therapy, and yes, at the heart of it all we have our clients do colonics! They are so important to the success of their treatments that we have our clients do them once every other day while in the 10 day treatment program! We treat all conditions and each and every treatment protocol our clients receive whether it be colitis to cancer, arthritis to arterial disease or Parkinson's to pain (anywhere), inflammation to immune issues, all have a gut health element which includes many colon hydrotherapies! I, personally, will not work with a person unless they agree to them because I work to win!

In comes Karin... the best colon hydrotherapist I have ever had the pleasure of working with. During her course work in naturopathic school, she quickly realized that no vitamin or mineral supplement or any new diet regiment or any other approach to improving health was going to work to the ultimate end of any measurable and sustainable success without thoroughly cleansing the colon which amounts to a life changing detoxification. It's an absolutely must. The years of dietary and other lifestyles that abuse and harm the body that brought you to your symptoms and discomfort are stuck in your gut in a tar-like matter called mucoid plaque. And in and around that there is likely a collection of yeast, fungus, mold, parasites, viruses, worms, harmful bacteria and even new bacterium growing from GMO (genetically modified) products which today are suspected in the case of BT corn which makes its own pesticide, is doing the same in your gut 24/7 eating away at the lining (possibly a key contributor to leaky gut). Some of the things I've seen come out of people in colon hydrotherapy sessions is horrifying!

Karin has always been my number-one choice for my own colonics as well as for my patients. She is knowledgeable beyond any colon hydrotherapist I've known, balanced in her views about health, has a comforting energy and is the most skilled therapist I've worked with.

I can't wait until her book is released as I know I'm going to get another chance to do my two favorite things... laugh and learn something new! And in her book, I'm sure I'll do a lot of both!

In service we shine,

Genita M. Mason H.H.P., N.C., F.E.
Medical Director
The Ozone Treatment Center

Acknowlegments

First, I'd like to thank my husband and wonderful children for supporting me and always being there, no matter what. Without them, I would never be able to do what I do best. My sister for her encouragement and pushing me to step outside my comfort zone, and to always believe in myself. My mom for teaching me that everything is possible, even when it seems impossible.

I want to thank each and every one of my clients along the way who have taught me so much about life and experience via the human connection.

I'm so happy I've been able to touch so many people's hearts and health and being a part of their lives. Last of all, I want to thank God for giving me the gift of embracing people with love.

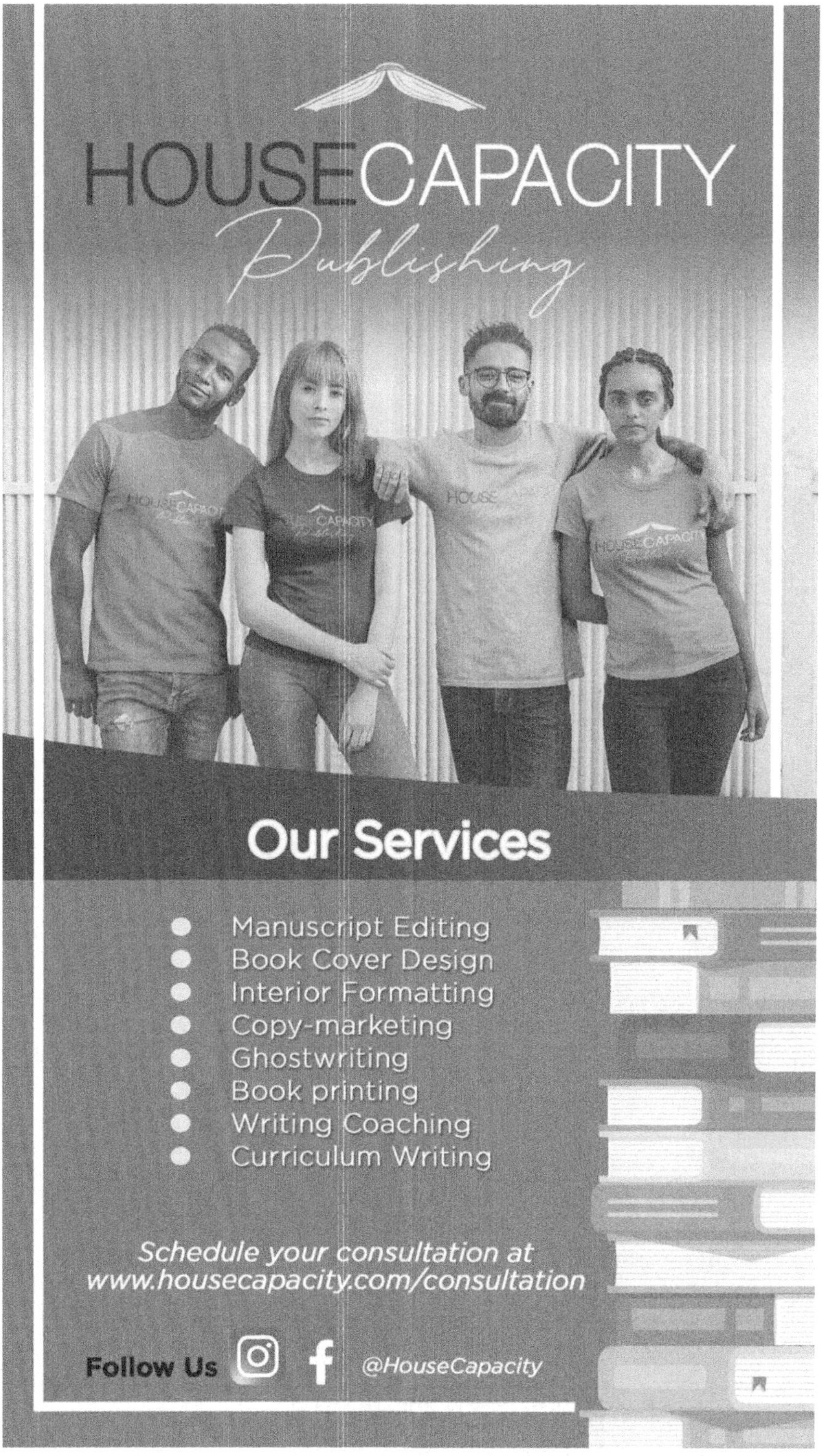
HOUSECAPACITY
Publishing
Our Services
Manuscript Editing
Book Cover Design
Interior Formatting
Copy-marketing
Ghostwriting
Book printing
Writing Coaching
Curriculum Writing
Schedule your consultation at
www.housecapacity.com/consultation
Follow Us
@HouseCapacity

Made in the USA
Middletown, DE
10 October 2022